THE ARMOR OF GOD
FITNESS & TRAINING
PROGRAM

THE KEY TO ULTIMATE
FITNESS FOR THE BODY OF CHRIST

PASTOR SHAOLIN MB ABRAMS, SR. PHD

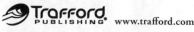

www.trafford.com

North America & international
toll-free: 1 888 232 4444 (USA & Canada)
phone: 250 383 6864 ♦ fax: 812 355 4082

THE ARMOR OF GOD

FITNESS & TRAINING PROGRAM

The Key To Ultimate Fitness For The Body Of Christ
**The Complete Guide & Training Manual For Physically Building
Through Fitness and Exercise *"THE BODY OF CHRIST"***

**Endurance
Strength
Power**

"Beloved, I pray above all things that you prosper and be in good health, even as your soul prospers." **(3 John 2)**

THE ARMOR OF GOD
FITNESS & TRAINING PROGRAM

This book is dedicated to my LORD & Savior Jesus Christ who is my personal and greatest hero of all times, and He has caused me through the Holy Spirit to write this training manual in hopes that the "True-Believer" in the Gospel of Jesus Christ would understand that as long as we are in the land of the living, we can enjoy the goodness of the Lord Through a healthy and fit lifestyle…because it was Christ who said that He has come to give us life and life more abundantly.

I would also like to rededicate this book to my mother because of the sacrifices that she has made for all her children and still making them for us today.

Thank you mom, for teaching me that without a personal relationship with the LORD and reverently fearing HIM, success is nothing because obedience is better than sacrifice.

"But without faith it is impossible to please HIM, for he who comes to GOD must believe that HE is, and that HE is a rewarder of those who diligently seek HIM."
(Hebrews 11:6)

THE ARMOR OF GOD

FITNESS & TRAINING PROGRAM

The Key To Ultimate Fitness For The Body Of Christ

First Edition Pyramid Fitness & The Armor of God Training 2004
Second Edition Pyramid Fitness & The Armor of God Training 2010

The Armor of God and colophon are registered trademarks of Pyramid Fitness & The Armor of God Training
Graphic designed by Gary@Epresso Courier & Printing, Inglewood CA

Manufactured in the United States of America

THE ARMOR OF GOD

FITNESS & TRAINING PROGRAM

PRESENTS

THE ARMOR OF GOD

Piece of Armor	Use	Application
Belt	Truth	Satan fights with lies, but sometimes his lies sound like truth and only those who believe in the Gospel of Jesus Christ can defeat Satan's lies with God's truth.
Breastplate	Righteousness	Satan often attacks our hearts; the seat of our emotions, self-worth and trust. God's righteousness is the breastplate that protects our hearts and ensures His approval. He loves us and sent His Son to die for us.
Footgear	Readiness to spread the Good News (*Gospel*)	Satan wants us to think that telling others the Good News (*Gospel*) is a worthless and hopeless task; and the size of task is too big and the negative responses are too much to handle. But the footgear God gives us is the motivation to continue to proclaim the true peace that is available in God; news everyone needs to hear.
Shield	Faith	What we see are Satan's attacks in the form of insults, setbacks, and temptations. With God's perspective, we can see beyond our circumstance and know that ultimate victory is ours.
Helmet	Salvation	Satan wants to make us doubt God, Jesus, and our salvation. The Helmet Protects our minds from doubting God's saving work in us.
Sword	The Word of God (*The Spirit)*	The sword is the only weapon of offense in this list of armor. There are times when we need to take the offensive against Satan. When we are tempted, we need to trust in the truth of God's Word.

THE ARMOR OF GOD

FITNESS & TRAINING PROGRAM

The premise of this training guide and manual is not based on workouts alone, but on educating the *Body of Christ* at large about the proper way to have life and life more abundantly according to God's Word. My entire adult life has been devoted to improving my *mind, body and spirit,* but the only way my *Life-Style* can be balanced is by ensuring that my *Immune System* protects me against any form of disease, *such as High Blood Pressure, Diabetes, Hypertension, High Cholesterol, etc.* Now, I don't claim that with this *Life-Style* change you will live any longer than the next person, but what I am attempting to convey is that with change you live *much healthier, have more energy, and be more alert to enjoy the many blessings that the LORD has promised in HIS Word!*

The reality is that you do not have to use steroids or muscle enhancing drugs *(steroid derivatives)* to achieve a great body, so stop listening to those *"so-called"* personal trainers who are just trying to sell you those expensive training sessions looking like they *eat cheeseburgers and french-fries for breakfast, lunch and dinner!* If a trainer's body does not appear as though he/she works out regularly or they look like they came straight out of a fitness magazine, *be careful because all that glitters isn't gold!* And it doesn't matter what that certificate says on their office wall, or how many hours of personal training time they have because when these *"so-called"* personal trainers tell you that they want to *"design a program specifically for you and your needs,"* ask yourself how in the world do they know it works if they have never tried it for themselves?

WE DON'T ASK A POOR MAN HOW TO GET RICH, SO BE WEARY OF THOSE WHO CANNOT DEMONSTRATE THEIR OWN CLAIMS!!!

THE ARMOR OF GOD

FITNESS & TRAINING PROGRAM

One of the first things to realize is that there are many different body types:

1. <u>Ectomorph:</u> Thin, flat chest, delicate build, young appearance, tall, lightly muscled, crouched shoulders, large brain, may have trouble gaining weight, and muscle growth takes longer.

2. <u>Mesomorph:</u> Hard, muscle body, overly mature appearance, rectangular shaped, thick skin, upright posture, gains or loses weight easily, and grows muscle quickly.

3. <u>Endomorph:</u> Soft body, underdeveloped muscles, rounded shaped, overdeveloped digestive system *(abdominals)*. Trouble losing weight, and generally gains muscle easily.

I realize that what I am about to say may offend some in the *Body of Christ,* but we need to stop listening to those doctors who have been telling us that there isn't any difference in ethnic body types and quit with the stereotypes because genetics does have a lot to do with the way a person is built and shaped. We will continue to be unhealthy if we try to obtain a suggested weight that has been obsolete for the past 35 years; and I don't know about you, but personally I am not trying to look like anyone on the cover of these *"so-called"* fitness magazines, starving myself and taking all kinds of diuretics just to have a *"six-pack!"*

The Word of God says that He shall supply all my needs, exceedingly and abundantly above all I ask for or even dream of, *food just happens to be one of those pleasures He has made available!*

THE ARMOR OF GOD

FITNESS & TRAINING PROGRAM

However, it is obvious that many of us have abused that pleasure, so with the inspiration of the Holy Spirit this training guide and manual has been written to help those in the *Body of Christ* get their eating habits back on the *"right track"* by first asserting that *"Dieting"* was meant for us to fail! We must get out of the habit of wanting to lose *"weight"* and start wanting to lose *"fat!"*

The Armor of God Fitness & Training Program consists of three *(3)* parts: *Endurance, Strength and Power.* I want you to understand that when you are building *Endurance* (Stamina), you also increase your *Strength and build Power.* Now, having *"Power"* doesn't mean that you will be able to lift the *"Empire State Building,"* but what it does mean is your muscles will respond in a situation that requires them to put forth more *strength* than usual *(e.g. If your child were involved in a life-threatening situation, you would need to utilize some "Power").*

The three *(3)* components of this program are broken down into three *(3)* different phases that consist of three *(3)* six *(6)* week periods, and as your body begins to adapt to the workout, you will notice a dramatic change in your *endurance* (stamina), and your *strength* will begin to increase as you start to gain *power to do all things through Christ Who gives you the strength and will strengthen you for the next eighteen* (18) *weeks.* Once you have completed all three *(3)* cycles, repeat the program; starting once again at *Endurance* and ending at *Power.*

THE ARMOR OF GOD
FITNESS & TRAINING PROGRAM

Muscle weighs more than fat, and for every five *(5)* pounds that you lose, three *(3)* pounds of muscle is lost, that's why all of those people who have lost a great deal of weight have a lot of excess skin hanging and have to get it surgically removed because the extra skin has no solid mass to hold its elasticity, and *without muscle to support our skin, we are left with human jelly!!* In this guide and training manual, I will give you straight-forward workout plans to fit your busy, and sometimes hectic lifestyles. *I will present an effective and real way to eat to live, rather than what you may be doing now, LIVING TO EAT!!* I won't sell you any false hopes or dreams, but if you commit to the eighteen *(18)* week fitness & training program that *I have laid out through the inspiration of the Holy Spirit,* you will not have any problems achieving your desired goals and dreams. Regardless of whether your goal is *toning, gaining mass, or achieving overall fitness,* when you make the decision to commit; *a change in your lifestyle takes place!!*

The Word of God says not to be conformed to this world, but be transformed by the renewing of your mind; and change begins in the MIND, *then the* BODY!!

The Armor of God Fitness & Training Program guide and manual will give you the ability to enhance your balance on all three *(3)* levels: Mentally *(GOD the Father),* Physically *(GOD the Son…Jesus Christ)* and Spiritually *(GOD the Holy Spirit).*

THE ARMOR OF GOD

FITNESS & TRAINING PROGRAM

One of the main reasons most people plateau with their workouts is because they never change or rotate their routine, but once a plateau is reached, individuals end up simply lifting weights without any physical benefits. Remember, for every five *(5)* pounds that you loose, three *(3)* pounds of muscle is lost, and we need muscle to keep the skin *tight and firm,* so you want to lose *fat* and not *muscle!* Do you think just because you spend hours using *cardio machines, aerobics, etc.* that you are losing the right type of weight, *because you may not be.* For the most part, during the first 20-30 minutes your body is burning nothing but *fat,* after that, *muscle and fat together!* And after a few weeks of all those *grueling machines and all that aerobic exercise,* you do lose some weight, but just how much *fat* have you really lost?

Don't be misled by all these *new-fangled gadgets* that claim to help you burn *fat, because they don't!* Understand that a man must have at least forty *(40)* grams of protein per meal and a woman must have twenty *(20)* grams of protein in order to maintain the muscle mass that you already have, but what will happen is that your body will get the proper *"food"* it needs in order to fuel itself, and this causes a chain reaction to make the body's *metabolism* speed up and burn *fat rather than muscle;* but once this starts happening, *your body will continue to burn fat twenty-four* (24) *hours a day, seven* (7) *days a week!*

THIS IS WHERE THE *"REAL"* WORKOUT BEGINS!!!

THE ARMOR OF GOD

FITNESS & TRAINING PROGRAM

The fitness & training program is numbered into days so that you can keep a steady workout going according to a suitable schedule; for example: *Instead of working out Monday-Friday or Tuesday-Saturday, Day One (1), for example would be Chest; Day Two (2), would be Back; Day Three (3), would be Legs; Day Four (4), would be Shoulders and Day Five (5) would be Arms* (Triceps & Biceps). This way, if you miss a day, you do not skip it, just continue with whatever day comes next. If you worked out on Monday and Tuesday *(Day One and Day Two),* then you missed *Wednesday,* just continue on *Thursday,* which would be *Day Three* (3). Remember to do abdominals everyday that you workout, *but do not use weights for the abs because like any other muscle they will grow thick and big!!* But the key to *hard, flat and defined abdominals are* isometrics, because they make your abs *hard and keep them tight* and when the fat is burned around your abs, they are left very well defined.

So with the help and inspiration of the Holy Spirit, I have designed *"The Armor of God Fitness & Training Program"* to benefit others; but more importantly, I myself have been using these principles for the past twenty-five *(25)* years and I know it works!!

This fitness and training program is very simple with basic movements, but in order to achieve optimal results, you must be *CONSISTENT!!* Remember, *its not how much weight you can lift, but the order in which you do your routine, and the proper form to get the desired results.* And whether you are trying to lose fat *(not weight),* gain lean muscle mass, or just tone up what you already have, you can achieve your goals with this program…*GUARANTEED!!!*

"For I can do everything through Christ who strengthens me and gives me strength." (**Philippians** 4:13)

"Beloved, I pray above all things that you may prosper and be in good health even as your soul prospers." (3 John 2)

THE ARMOR OF GOD

FITNESS & TRAINING PROGRAM

NOW THAT WE HAVE TAKEN CARE OF THE FUNDAMENTALS, LETS'S BEGIN:

Phase One: Endurance – Six (6) Weeks

The Word of God says; "The race wasn't given to the swift or the strong, but to those who <u>endure</u> to the end." (1 Cor. 9:24)

Five (5) days on, and Two (2) days off. One (1) body part per day.

Take three (3) deep breaths in between each set. Make sure you drink plenty of water after each set. The larger muscle groups require more work; that's why we do twenty (20) sets for the major muscle groups *(chest, back, legs, and shoulders)*, and 15 sets for the smaller muscles *(triceps, hamstrings, and calves)*, you need less work because you can't train a major muscle without training the smaller muscle indirectly.

<u>For example:</u> When you train your <u>chest</u> *(major muscle)*, you also train your triceps *(smaller muscle)* at the same time. Training your <u>back</u> *(major muscle)*, you also train your <u>biceps</u> *(smaller muscle)*. When you train your <u>quads</u> *(major muscle)*, you also train your <u>hamstrings and calves</u> *(smaller muscle)*. That's why only fifteen *(15)* sets are necessary for the smaller muscles because we do not want to over-train them.

THE ARMOR OF GOD

FITNESS & TRAINING PROGRAM

Day One (1)—Cardio, Chest & Abs

Cardio – 30 Minutes *(Treadmill)*

1. Set control on Manual

2. Enter your Weight

3. Enter the Incline (8.0 + Enter)

4. Enter the Time (30 minutes)

5. Enter your Speed (Will be determined)

To determine your initial speed, start off with a speed comfortable with you, and every five (5) minutes increase your speed by point one (.1), for example: 2.1 becomes 2.2 at the five (5) minute interval, 2.2 becomes 2.3 at the ten (10) minute interval, 2.3 becomes 2.4 at the fifteen (15) minute interval, 2.4 becomes 2.5 at the twenty (20) minute interval, and 2.5 becomes 2.6 at the twenty-five (25) minute interval and that would be the last time you increased your speed. Once you go into the "Cool Down" position (This is an extra five (5) minute process), the incline and your speed starts to drop down every minute, but watch your speed because you don't want it to drop past the speed in which you started with.

Do this for the entire week and then following week, you increase your incline to 9.0, and start at the speed you start with the previous week. Repeat this until you have reached the 15.0 level on the incline. To calculate how many calories you have burned each week, you take what you burned that day by how many times a week you do cardio (treadmill).

THE ARMOR OF GOD

FITNESS & TRAINING PROGRAM

For example: If you burned four hundred (400) calories each day for five (5) days, would be 400 x 5 = 2000 calories per week, etc.

Tip: Always remember that you burn more fat by walking (treadmill) then by running or jogging because walking is the only <u>true</u> way to burn nothing but <u>fat.</u>

<u>Chest</u> – Five (5) sets, Fifteen (15) reps w/increase in weight for each set

<u>*Incline Bench Press (Barbell)*</u>

Lying flat on the bench, keeping your back straight and your buttocks firmly against the seat, place your hands on the outside lines on the bar for proper positioning. Next, lift the bar off the rack and lower it so the bar touches the bottom of your neck and the upper part of your chest.

Next, do five (5) sets of fifteen (15) reps w/<u>increase</u> in weight until you can no longer do the fifteen (15) reps, but do not go lower than ten (10) reps. Then <u>decrease</u> weight back down to be able to get the fifteen (15) reps that are necessary.

<u>*Decline Bench Press (Barbell)*</u>

For proper positioning of your body, sit down on the bench and place your feet underneath the pads on the front of the bench. Lying flat on your back, place your hands on the outside lines of the bar and then lift the bar off the rack. Lower the bar down towards your chest so it touches the bottom of your chest and the tops of your abs. Next, do five (5) sets of fifteen (15) reps w/increase in weight until you can no longer do the fifteen (15) reps, but do not go lower than ten (10) reps. Then decrease weight back down to be able to get the fifteen (15) reps that are necessary.

THE ARMOR OF GOD

FITNESS & TRAINING PROGRAM

Incline Press (Hammer-Strength)

Adjust the seat and raising your arms shoulder-height, making sure that the bar touches your shoulders. For the proper positioning of your hands, place your thumbs at the tip of the rubber on the bar, now stretch out your thumb and grip the bar; and pushing the bar forward, do five (5) sets of fifteen (15) reps w/<u>increase</u> in weight until you can no longer do the fifteen (15) reps, but do not go lower than ten (10) reps. Then <u>decrease</u> weight back down to be able to get the fifteen (15) reps that necessary.

Decline Press (Hammer-Strength)

Adjust the seat and sit back so the bar is going across the middle part of your chest. For the proper positioning of your hands, place your thumbs at the tip of the rubber on the bar and stretch them out to grip the bar. Pushing the bar forward, do five (5) sets of fifteen (15) reps w/<u>increase</u> in weight until you can no longer do the fifteen (15) reps, but do not go lower than ten (10) reps. Then <u>decrease</u> weight back down to be able to get the fifteen (15) reps that are necessary.

Abdominals (Upper, Middle, and Lower)

Day One (1) – Upper Abs

<u>Flat Crunches – Two (2) sets, Twenty-five (25) reps per set</u>

Laying flat on your back with your legs straight out, cross your left leg over your right leg, and place your arms across your chest as though you were hugging yourself. Now try to find a spot on the ceiling you can focus on and raise up just enough so your shoulders come off the floor; do this twenty-five (25) times, take three (3) deep breaths, switch your legs and repeat this twenty-five (25) more times. Take three (3) more deep breaths and go to the next exercise.

THE ARMOR OF GOD

FITNESS & TRAINING PROGRAM

Heel Crunches – One (1) set, Twenty-five (25) reps per set

Laying flat on your back, bend your legs so your heels are almost touching your buttocks, and place your arms across your chest as though you were hugging yourself. Now try to find a spot on the ceiling you can focus on and raise up just enough so your shoulders come off the floor; do this twenty-five (25) times, take three (3) deep breaths and go to the next exercise.

Twist Crunches – Two (2) sets, Twenty-five (25) reps per set

Laying flat on your back, bend your legs so your heels are almost touching your buttocks; then take your left leg and place it across your right knee.

Place your right are behind your head and your left arm across your ribcage. Now rise up as though you were doing a crunch and bend yourself sideways towards your left foot, do this twenty-five (25) times.

Take three (3) deep breaths, switch sides and repeat this twenty-five (25) more times. Take three (3) more deep breaths and go to the next exercise.

"L" Crunches – One (1) set Twenty-five (25) reps per set

Laying flat on your back, lift your legs so your body forms the letter "L"; then place your arms across your chest as though you were hugging yourself.

Next, find a focus point on the ceiling and rise up just enough so your shoulders come up off the floor; do this twenty-five (25) times and then take three (3) deep breaths and go to the next exercise.

THE ARMOR OF GOD

FITNESS & TRAINING PROGRAM

Pyramid Crunches – One (1) set, Twenty-five (25) reps per set

Laying flat on your back, raise your legs up and at the same time, bring your arms toward them making a "Pyramid *(Triangle)*" while lifting your shoulders off of the floor. Make sure you are bringing both legs and arms up together; do this twenty-five (25) times, then take three (3) deep breaths and go to the next exercise.

Side Bend Crunches – Two (2), Twenty-five (25) reps per set

Laying flat on your back, twist your body so your bottom leg is straight and your top leg goes into the back of your knee, forming the number four (4). Place both your shoulders flat on the floor and put both your arms behind your neck. Find a focus point on the ceiling and rise up just enough so your shoulders come off of the floor, but this time, you must keep yourself from twisting towards the side that your legs are pointing by coming up as straight as possible. Do these twenty-five (25) times, take three (3) deep breaths, switch sides, and then repeat exercise.

Day Two (2) – Middle Abs

Standing Twists w/Stick – One (1) set, One Hundred (100) reps per set

Standing with legs firmly planted and shoulder-width apart, place stick *(pole)* comfortably on the back of your neck so when you twist, it's not resting on your shoulders. Keeping a firm position with your body, with your head straight and eyes forward, twist your body so only your upper body *(torso)* twists from the side position to the front position. Remember not to allow your lower body to move, nor your head; then twist the stick *(pole)* on both sides until it makes a complete circle and the ends of the bar faces directly in front of you.

Do one hundred (100) reps on each side for a total of two hundred (200) reps; take three (3) deep breaths and go on to the next exercise.

THE ARMOR OF GOD

FITNESS & TRAINING PROGRAM

Standing Twists w/Stick Extended – Two (2) sets, Twenty-five (25) reps per set

Standing with legs firmly planted and shoulder-width apart, take the stick *(pole)* and extend it so it's straight ahead of you, shoulder-height. Starting from the left side, twist yourself as far as you can, keeping the stick *(pole)* back to the front, and <u>don't</u> twist yourself to the other side because you <u>must</u> stop the bar right in front of you. Do these twenty-five (25) times, take three (3) deep breaths switch and then repeat the exercise.

Standing Side-Bends w/Stick Overhead Two (2) sets, Twenty-five (25) reps per set

Stand with your legs firmly planted and shoulder-width apart, take the stick *(pole)* and raise it almost above your head so when you look up at it, it's right at eye level. Starting on the left side, bend your upper body *(torso)* so the stick *(pole)* is the floor in a vertical position and then bring it back to where you started, but <u>don't</u> go past the starting point. Do these twenty-five (25) times, take three (3) deep breaths, switch sides and repeat the exercise.

Day Three (3) – Lower Abs

Standing Side Twist – One (1) set, Twenty-five (25) reps per set

Stand with your legs firmly planted and shoulder-width apart; keep a firm position with your lower body while keeping your head straight and your eyes forward. Now raise your arms up, shoulder-height and twist your body so only your upper body *(torso)* twists from the side position to the front. Remember not to allow your lower body to move while keeping your head forward. Keeping your arms up, twist your body from side to side so your hands come to the front of you and once your hands have completed a full rotation, that's one (1) rep. Do these

THE ARMOR OF GOD

FITNESS & TRAINING PROGRAM

twenty-five (25) times, take three (3) deep breaths and go on to the next exercise.

Windmills – One (1) set, Twenty-five (25) reps per set

Standing with legs firmly planted on the floor, position your feet so they're open enough so you can touch the floor comfortably. Place your hands on your hips, then take your left hand and touch your right foot, then come back to your starting position; and placing your hands back on your hips, take your right hand and touch your left foot. Come back up and place your hands back on your hips. Do these twenty-five (25) times, take three (3) deep breaths; then go on to the next exercise.

Standing Leg Twists – One (1) set, Twenty-five (25) reps per set

Standing with legs firmly planted and shoulder-width apart crossing your arms and bringing your left knee up, twist it towards your right elbow. Next, take your right knee and twist it up toward your left elbow; then do these twenty-five (25) times, take three (3) deep breaths and go on to the next exercise.

Tic-Tocs – One (1) set, Twenty-five (25) reps per set

Standing with legs firmly planted and shoulder-width apart raise your arms up so they're in an upright position. Bending towards your left side, point your right hand straight so your left hand is also pointing towards the floor. Come back to an upright position, bend towards the right side while pointing your left hand up and your right hand points toward the floor; then come back to an upright position; do these twenty-five (25) times.

THE ARMOR OF GOD

FITNESS & TRAINING PROGRAM

Always remember to do abs everyday and rotate whichever one you have
not done; for example: If you do the upper abs on day one (1), then on
day two (2), you do the middle, and on day three (3) you do the lower abs.
But on day four (4) you go back to the upper abs, and then on day five (5)
finish with the middle abs.

Day Two (2)—Cardio, Back & Abs

Cardio – 30 Minutes (Treadmill)

See example in day one (1)

Back – Five (5) sets, Fifteen (15) reps w/increase in weight for each set

T-Bar Rows (Hammer-Strength)

For proper positioning of your body, stand firmly with your feet place
so the strongest is in the front of the other. Next, place your hands at
the very end of the rubber on the bar, now pull the bar as close to you as
possible without hitting the bench and do five (5) sets of fifteen (15) reps
w/<u>increase</u> in weight until you can no longer do the fifteen (15) reps, but
do not go lower than ten (10) reps. Then <u>decrease</u> weight back down to be
able to get the fifteen (15) reps that are necessary.

Low-Pulley Rows (Hammer-Strength)

Adjust your seat so when you sit down, your chin can touch the top part
of the seat. For the proper positioning of your hands, place your hands
on the bottom half of the curve on the bar. As you pull the weight
towards you, sit up straight in the seat so your chest is flat against it and
do five (5) sets of fifteen (15) reps w/<u>increase</u> in weight until you can no
longer do the fifteen (15) reps, but do not go lower than ten (10) reps.
Then <u>decrease</u> weight back down to be able to get the fifteen (15) reps
that are necessary.

THE ARMOR OF GOD

FITNESS & TRAINING PROGRAM

Bent-Over Rows (Barbell)

For proper positioning of your hands, place them on the outside lines of the bar, and then standing with your feet shoulder-width apart, bend at your waist and pull the weight towards your stomach and do five (5) sets of fifteen (15) reps w/<u>increase</u> in weight until you can no longer do the fifteen (15) reps, but do not go lower than ten (10) reps. Then <u>decrease</u> weight back down to be able to get the fifteen (15) reps that are necessary.

Seated Cable Rows (Cable Machine)

Attach V-Shaped bar to the cable line, and place your feet so they are just a little bit below your knees about shoulder-width apart. Bringing the V-Shape bar to your stomach, do five (5) sets of fifteen (15) reps w/ <u>increase</u> in weight until you can no longer do the fifteen (15) reps, but do not go lower than ten (10) reps. Then <u>decrease</u> weight back down to be able to get the fifteen (15) reps that are necessary.

Abdominals (Upper, Middle, and Lower)

Always remember to do abs everyday and rotate whichever one you have not done; for example: If you do the upper abs on day one (1), then on day two (2), you do the middle, and on day three (3) you the lower abs. But on day four (4) you go back to the upper abs, and then on day five (5) finish with the middle abs.

Day Three (3) – Cardio, Legs (Quads, Hamstrings & Calves), and Abs

Cardio – 30 Minutes (Treadmill)

See example in day one (1)

Quads – Five (5) sets, Fifteen (15) reps w/increase in weight for each set

THE ARMOR OF GOD

FITNESS & TRAINING PROGRAM

Squats (Barbell)

Go underneath the bar and place your neck evenly between the openings on the bar. After doing this, place your hands on the lines of the bar to balance it once you have lifted it from its position. Using your legs, push up and take two (2) steps backward so you will clear the rack and have no difficulty squatting.

For the proper positioning of your feet, place them shoulder-width apart so you can distribute your weight evenly. Next, do five (5) sets of fifteen (15) reps w/<u>increase</u> in weight until you can no longer so the fifteen (15) reps, but do not go lower than ten (10) reps. Then <u>decrease</u> weight back down to be able to get the fifteen (15) reps that are necessary.

Seated Incline Leg Press (Hammer-Strength)

For proper positioning of your feet, place your feet shoulder-width apart so they are touching the very top part of the machine. Bringing your legs down so they touch your chest, do five (5) sets of fifteen (15) reps w/ <u>increase</u> in weight until you can no longer do the fifteen (15) reps, but do not go lower than ten (10) reps. Then <u>decrease</u> weight back down to be able to get the fifteen (15) reps that are necessary.

Hack Squats (Hammer-Strength)

For proper positioning of your body, adjust yourself so the pads fit comfortably on your shoulders and then place your feet should-width apart so they are touching the very top part of the machine. Next, lower yourself down as though you were sitting; do five (5) sets of fifteen (15) reps w/<u>increase</u> in weight until you can no longer do the fifteen (15) reps, but do not go lower than ten (10) reps. Then <u>decrease</u> weight back down to be able to get the fifteen (15) reps that are necessary.

THE ARMOR OF GOD

FITNESS & TRAINING PROGRAM

Leg Extensions (Leg Machine)

For proper positioning of your feet, place your feet shoulder-width apart and placing them underneath the pad at the bottom of machine. Next, bring legs up so they come to a vertical position and do five (5) sets of fifteen (15) reps w/<u>increase</u> in weight until you can no longer do the fifteen (15) reps, but do not go lower than ten (10) reps. Then <u>decrease</u> weight back down to be able to get the fifteen (15) reps that are necessary.

Hamstrings – Five (5) sets, Fifteen (15) reps w/increase in weight for each set

Leg Curls (Hammer-Strength)

Lying flat on your stomach, place your legs underneath the pad at the end of the machine so your heels fit comfortably on the pad. Next, bring your legs up so they touch the back of your buttocks and do five (5) sets of fifteen (15) reps w/<u>increase</u> in weight until you can no longer do the fifteen (15) reps, but do not go lower than ten (10) reps. Then <u>decrease</u> weight back down to be able to get the fifteen (15) reps that are necessary.

<u>Calves – *Five (5) sets of Fifteen (15) reps w/increase in weight for each set*</u>

Standing Calf Raises (Calf Machine)

For proper positioning of your body, place your shoulders comfortably between the pads on the machine and then for the proper positioning of your feet, place them shoulder-width apart so most of your foot is on the rubber pad. Keeping your knees locked, lower your heels so the toes on your feet stick straight up as you raise up on your feet; and make sure that they are in a flat position before you raise completely to the top as far as you can on the balls of your feet. Next, do five (5) sets of fifteen (15) reps w/<u>increase</u> in weight until you

THE ARMOR OF GOD

FITNESS & TRAINING PROGRAM

can no longer do the fifteen (15) reps, but do not go lower than ten (10) reps. Then <u>decrease</u> weight back down to be able to get the fifteen (15) reps that are necessary.

Abdominals (Upper, Middle & Lower)

Always remember to do abs everyday and rotate whichever one you have not done, for example: *If you do the upper abs on day one (1), then on day two (2), you do the middle, and on day three (3) you do the lower abs. But on day four (4) you go back to the upper abs, and then on day five (5) finish with the middle abs.*

Day Four (4) – Cardio, Shoulders, and Abs

Cardio – 30 Minutes (Treadmill)

See example in day one (1)

Shoulders – Five (5) sets, Fifteen (15) reps w/increase in weight for each set

Seated Shoulder Press (Hammer-Strength)

Adjust the seat so bar is even with the top part of your chest, and then sit down with your back firmly against the seat so your back is straight. For proper positioning of your hands, place thumbs at the tip of the rubber in the bar and stretch them out to grip the bar. Pushing upward, do five (5) sets of fifteen (15) reps w/<u>increase</u> in weight until you can no longer do the fifteen (15) reps, but do not go lower than ten (10) reps. Then <u>decrease</u> weight back down to be able to get the fifteen (15) reps that are necessary.

THE ARMOR OF GOD

FITNESS & TRAINING PROGRAM

Shoulder Shrugs (Barbell)

For proper positioning of your body, stand so you are evenly between the open spaces on the bar; and then position your hands so your grip is even with the outside of your legs. Next, place your chin on your chest, keeping your arms firmly at your side, lifting up your shoulders as far as they can go. Do five (5) sets of fifteen (15) reps w/<u>increase</u> in weight until you can no longer do the fifteen (15) reps, but do not go lower than ten (10) reps. Then <u>decrease</u> weight back down to be able to get the fifteen (15) reps that are necessary.

Side Lateral Raises (Dumbbells)

For proper positioning of your body, stand with your feet shoulder-width apart as you hold the dumbbells against your body, and begin to raise them so they are stretched out evenly with your shoulders. Next, do five (5) sets of fifteen (15) reps w/<u>increase</u> in weight until you can no longer do the fifteen (15) reps, but do not go lower than ten (10) reps. Then <u>decrease</u> weight back down to be able to get the fifteen (15) reps that are necessary.

Rear Delt Flyes (Dumbbells)

For proper positioning of your body, stand with your feet shoulder-width apart as you hold the dumbbells against your body, and bend your body at the waist so your arms are stretched out evenly with your shoulders. Lower your arms so that the dumbbells touch and then do five (5) sets of fifteen (15) reps w/increase in weight until you can no longer do the fifteen (15) reps, but do not go lower than ten (10) reps. Then decrease weight back down to be able to get the fifteen (15) reps that are necessary.

THE ARMOR OF GOD

FITNESS & TRAINING PROGRAM

Abdominals (Upper, Middle, and Lower)

Always remember to do abs everyday and rotate whichever one you have not done, for example: If you do the upper abs on day one (1), then on day two (2) you do the middle, and on day three (3) you do the lower abs. But on day four (4), you go back to the upper abs and then on day five (5) finish with lower abs.

Day Five (5) – Cardio, Arms (Triceps & Biceps), and Abs

Cardio – 30 Minutes (Treadmill)

See example in day one (1)

Triceps – Five (5) sets, Fifteen (15) reps w/increase in weight for each set

Close-Grip Bench Press (Barbell)

Laying down flat on your back, place your hands on each side of the bar where the grooves begin. Next, lift the bar off the rack and bring it down to the bottom edge of your chest. Push out so the bar is moving forward, and do five (5) sets of fifteen (15) reps w/<u>increase</u> in weight until you can no longer do the fifteen (15) reps, but do not go lower than ten (10) reps. Then <u>decrease</u> weight back down to be able to get the fifteen (15) reps that are necessary.

Triceps Extensions (EZ Curl Bar)

Laying flat on your back, grip the curl bar in the middle on the inside of the curve. Slide down so the back of your head touches the bench and you can look right in front of you. Next, place the bar on your chin and then do five (5) sets of fifteen (15) reps w/<u>same</u> weight for each set.

THE ARMOR OF GOD

FITNESS & TRAINING PROGRAM

Set One (1): Start at the chin

Set Two (2): Go to the bridge of nose

Set Three (3): Go to the forehead

Set Four (4): At the back of the head

Set Five (5): Start at the back of the head and push out

Triceps Pull-Downs (Cable Machine)

First, place the small, straight triceps bar onto the cable. For proper positioning of hands, place them at the very ends of the bar gripping it. Next, place your feet shoulder-width apart so you can distribute your weight evenly while pulling the weight towards you. Keeping the cable line in front of you *(actually looking at it)*, and keeping the cable close to your body; pull the cable down towards the floor until you have totally stretched out your arms. As the bar goes back up to its original position, make sure that your arms only come up to a "L" position or slightly underneath the lower part of your chest. Repeat this for five (5) sets of fifteen (15) reps w/<u>increase</u> in weight until you can no longer do the fifteen (15) reps, but do not go lower than ten (10) reps. Then <u>decrease</u> weight back down to be able to get the fifteen (15) reps that are necessary.

Biceps – Five (5) sets, Fifteen (15) reps w/increase in weight for each set

Standing Barbell Curls (Barbell)

For proper positioning of your feet, stand shoulder-width apart and place your hands on the outside lines of the bar for proper grip. Next, raise the bar so it reaches your chin without you lowering your head; then do five (5) sets of fifteen (15) reps, w/<u>increase</u> in weight

THE ARMOR OF GOD

FITNESS & TRAINING PROGRAM

until you can no longer do the fifteen (15) reps, but do not go lower than ten (10) reps. Then <u>decrease</u> weight back down to be able to get the fifteen (15) reps that are necessary.

<u>Seated Barbell Curls (Hammer-Strength)</u>

Adjust seat, then place your arms over the bench with your armpits on top of the pad making your arms stretch forward. For proper positioning of your hands, grip the attached bar where the rubber ends; then pull the bar so it reaches your face. Do five (5) sets of fifteen (15) reps w/<u>increase</u> in weight until you can no longer do the fifteen (15) reps, but do not go lower than ten (10) reps. Then <u>decrease</u> weight back down to be able to get the fifteen (15) reps that are necessary.

<u>Seated Concentration Curls (Cable Machine)</u>

Adjust cable pulley down to the last position on the machine. Attach the short straight-bar to the cable, and stretch out your arms so the weights stay down and your arms are as straight as they can go. Next, for proper positioning of your body, squat down and find a comfortable stance for your feet; stretching, place your armpits on top of your knees. Now sit down so you have complete balance, pulling the bar towards the front of your face and do five (5) sets of fifteen (15) reps w/ <u>increase</u> in weight until you can no longer do the fifteen (15) reps, but do not go lower than ten (10) reps. Then <u>decrease</u> weight back down to be able to get the fifteen (15) reps that are necessary.

THE ARMOR OF GOD

FITNESS & TRAINING PROGRAM

Abdominals (Upper, Middle, and Lower)

Always remember to do abs everyday and rotate whichever one you have not done, for example: If you do the upper abs on day one (1) then on day two (2) you do the middle, and on day three (3) you do the lower abs. But on day four (4) you go back to the upper abs and then on day five (5) finish with lower abs.

Phase Two: Strength – Six (6) Weeks

The Word of God says; "I can do all things through Christ Who gives me the <u>strength</u> and <u>strengthens</u> me." (Phil. 4:13)

Four (4) days on, three (3) days off. Two (2) body parts per day, with two (2) to three (3) minutes rest in between each set.

Two (2) different exercises per body part in a pyramid; for example: Five (5) sets for each exercise up w/<u>increase</u> in weight until the last set is reached in the series of major muscles (chest, back, legs and shoulders). Then do five (5) sets for each exercise (3 exercises per set) up w/<u>increase</u> in weight until the last set is reached in the series of minor muscles (triceps, biceps, hamstrings and calves) as you did with the major muscles.

Do five (5) sets for each exercise w/<u>increase</u> in weight with each set, doing ten (10) reps for each set.

Once you can not get ten (10) reps, don't drop below eight (8) reps; then decrease the weights so that you can get ten (10) reps. *Repeat formula for next set of exercises* (triceps, biceps, hamstrings and calves).

THE ARMOR OF GOD

FITNESS & TRAINING PROGRAM

On your first set, you must be able to get the initial ten; then on your next set, if you only get eight (8) that's okay because now you have a goal to reach for.

Just decrease your weight back down so you can get your ten (10) reps.

Always make sure you drink plenty of water after each set.

Day One (1) – Cardio, Chest, Biceps and Abs

Cardio – 30 Minutes (Treadmill)

See example in phase one (1), day one (1)

Chest – Five (5) sets, of ten (10) reps w/increase in weight for each set

Incline Bench Press (Barbell)

Lying firmly on the bench with your back straight and your buttocks seated flatly, place your hands on the outside lines on the bar for proper positioning. Next, lift the bar off the rack and lower it so the bar touches the bottom of your neck and upper part of your chest.

Do five (5) sets of ten (10) reps w/<u>increase</u> in weight for each set.

Decline Bench Press (Barbell)

For proper positioning of your body, sit down and place your feet underneath the pads on the front of the bench and lie down so your head is even with the end of the bench. Next, grip the bar on the outside of the lines and then lift the bar off the rack and lower it so the bar touches the bottom of your chest and the top of your abs.

THE ARMOR OF GOD

FITNESS & TRAINING PROGRAM

Do five (5) sets of ten (10) reps w/<u>increase</u> in weight for each set.

Incline Bench Press (Dumbbell)

For proper positioning of the bench, adjust bench to the first position, and then grip the dumbbells firmly in your hands. Next, lie down and bring the dumbbells to your chest. Do five (5) sets of ten (10) reps w/<u>increase</u> in weight for each set.

Decline Bench Press (Hammer-Strength)

For proper positioning of seat, adjust it so when you sit down on the seat and raise your arms up, the bar touches your shoulders evenly. Next, using your thumbs as a guide, place them at the very end of the bar where the rubber begins and extend your hand as to get a measurement. As you push the bar forward, make sure your back is firmly against the seat. Do five (5) sets ten of (10) reps w/<u>increase</u> in weight for each set.

Biceps – Five (5) sets, of ten (10) reps w/increase in weight for each set

Standing Barbell Curls (Barbell)

For proper positioning of your feet, stand with your feet shoulder-width apart and place your hands on the outside line of the barbell for the proper grip; and then bring the bar up towards your chin. Do five (5) sets of ten (10) reps w/<u>increase</u> in weight for each set.

Seated Barbell Curls (Hammer-Strength)

After adjusting your seat, place your arms over the bench, so your armpits are on top of the pad making your arms stretch forward. Next, for proper positioning of your hands; grip the attached bar where the

THE ARMOR OF GOD

FITNESS & TRAINING PROGRAM

rubber ends, and then pull bar so it reaches your face. Do five (5) sets of ten (10) reps w/<u>increase</u> in weight for each set.

Seated Concentration Curls (Cable Machine)

Adjust cable pulley down to the last position on the machine. Attach the short straight-bar to the cable, and then stretch out your arms so the weights stay down and your arms are as straight as they can go.

For proper positioning of your body, squat down and find a comfortable stance for your feet, then stretch and place your armpits on top of your knees.

Sitting down and balance yourself, pulling the bar towards the front of your face. Do five (5) sets of ten (10) reps w/<u>increase</u> in weight for each set.

Abdominals (Upper, Middle and Lower)

Always remember to do abs everyday and rotate whichever on you have not done; for example: If you do the upper abs on day one (1) then on day two (2) do the middle, and on day three (3) the lower abs. But on day four (4), go back to the upper abs and on day five (5) finish with lower abs.

Tip: Any weight you can do for ten (10) reps or more is considered a warm-up set because all you are trying to do is bring blood to the muscle you are working, but oftentimes we do too many warm-ups and have nothing left for the actual workout.

Day Two (2) – Cardio, Legs (Quads & Calves) and Abs

Cardio – 30 Minutes (Treadmill)

See example in phase one (1), day one (1)

THE ARMOR OF GOD

FITNESS & TRAINING PROGRAM

Quads – Five (5) sets, of ten (10) reps w/increase in weight for each set

Squats (Barbell)

Go underneath the bar and place your neck evenly between the openings on the bar. After doing this, place your hands on the outside lines of the bar so you can balance it on your shoulders. Using your legs, push up and take a couple of steps backward so you can clear the rack without having any trouble squatting. For proper positioning of your feet, place them shoulder-width apart so you can distribute your weight evenly; do five (5) sets of ten (10) reps w/<u>increase</u> in weight for each set.

Incline Leg Press (Hammer-Strength)

For proper positioning of the seat, adjust it to the last position on the bench until it's almost flat; then sit down and lie flat on your back. Place your feet shoulder-width apart so they are touching the very top part of the machine and bring your legs down so they touch your chest. Do five (5) sets of ten (10) reps w/<u>increase</u> in weight for each set.

Hack Squats (Hammer-Strength)

For proper positioning of your body, adjust yourself so the pads fit comfortably on your shoulders; then place your feet shoulder-width apart so they are touching the very top of the machine. Next, lower yourself down as though you were going to sit. Do five (5) sets ten (10) reps w/ <u>increase</u> in weight for each set.

Seated Leg Extensions (Leg Machine)

For proper positioning of your feet, place your feet shoulder-width apart and place them underneath the pad at the bottom of the machine.

Next, bring your legs up so they come to a vertical position and holding the weight for three (3) seconds so legs are contracted to their fullest

THE ARMOR OF GOD

FITNESS & TRAINING PROGRAM

Day Three(3)-Back & Triceps and Abs

Cardio – 30 Minutes (Treadmill)

See example in phase one (1), day one (1)
Back - Five (5) sets, of ten (10) reps w/increase in weight for each set

Low Pulley Rows (Hammer-Strength)

Adjust your seat so when you sit down, your chin can touch the top part of the seat. For proper positioning of your hands, place them on the bottom half of the curve on the bar. As you pull the weight towards you, sit up straight in the seat so your chest is flat against it and do five (5) sets of ten (10) reps w/increase in weight for each set.

Bent-Over Rows (Hammer-Strength)

For proper positioning of your hands, place them on the outside lines of the bar, and for proper positioning of your feet, stand shoulder-width apart; bend over so your body forms the letter "L". Next, pull the weight towards your stomach, and then do five (5) sets ten (10) reps w/increase in weight for each set.

Seated Cable Rows (Cable Machine)

For proper positioning of the machine, attach the V-Shaped bar to the cable and then adjust the seat so your legs are just below your waist. Gripping the V-Shaped bar in your hands, pull it towards your waist as you stick out your chest, and then do five (5) sets ten (10) reps w/increase in weight for each set.

Triceps - Five (5) sets, of ten (10) reps w/increase in weight for each set

Close-Grip Bench Press (Barbell)

Lying down flat on the bench, place your hands on each side of the bar where the groves begin. Next, lift the bar off the rack and bring it down to the bottom edge of your chest. Push the bar out so it's moving forward, and then do five (5) sets of ten (10) reps w/increase in weight for each set.

Triceps Extensions (EZ Curl Bar)

Lying down flat on the bench, grip the curl bar in the middle on the inside of the curve. Slide down so the back of your head touches the bench and you can look right in front of you. Next, do five (5) sets of ten (10) reps w/ same weight for each set.

Set One (1): Start at the chin.
Set Two (2): Go to the eyes.
Set Three (3): Go to the forehead.
Set Four (4): Go to the back of the head.
Set Five (5): Start at the back of the head, and push the weight outward.

Triceps Pull-Downs (Cable Machine)

Place the V-Shaped bar on the cable, and for proper positioning of your feet, stand shoulder-width apart and grip the bar all the way at the end. Pull cable down so your arms are fully extended and as the weight takes your arms back up, stop as they form the letter "L", and then do five (5) sets of ten (10) reps w/increase in weight until you cannot get 10 reps, and then decrease the weight back down to get 10 reps.

Abdominals (Upper, Middle and Lower)

Always remember to do abs everyday and rotate whichever one you have not done; example: If you do the upper abs on day one (1) then on day two (2) do the middle and on day three (3) do the lower abs; but on day four (4) go back and do the upper abs, finishing off with lower abs on day five (5).

Day Four (4)-Shoulders & Hamstrings and Abs
Cardio – 30 Minutes (Treadmill) See example in phase one (1), day one (1)
Shoulders - Five (5) sets, of ten (10) reps w/increase in weight for each set

Seated Shoulder Press (Hammer-Strength)

Adjust the seat so that the bar is even with the top part of your chest and then sit down with your back firmly against the seat so your back is straight. For proper positioning of your hands, place thumbs at the tip of the rubber on the bar and stretch them out to grip the bar. Pushing upward, do five (5) sets of ten (10) reps w/increase in weight for each set.

Standing Shoulder Shrugs (Barbell)

For proper positioning of your body, stand so that you are evenly between the open spaces on the bar. Next, position your hands so your grip is even with the outside of your legs, and then place your chin on your chest, keeping your arms firmly at your side. Now lift your shoulders as to say "I don't know," then do five (5) sets of ten (10) reps w/increase in weight for each set.

Seated Shoulder Press (Dumbbells)

For proper positioning of your body, sit so your back is straight and your buttocks are firmly against the seat, and then gripping the dumbbells firmly in your hands, place them on your legs so you can position yourself to lift them. Next, bring the dumbbells to your shoulders with them pointing forward and pushing upward, bring the dumbbells together and then do five (5) sets of ten (10) reps w/increase in weight for each set.

Seated Rear-Delt Flyes (Hammer-Strength)

For proper positioning of them machine, adjust the seat so you are sitting with your chest against the seat, and your chin on the top of the pad. Next, adjust the machine to the last forward position, and gripping the ends of the rubber on the bar, open your arms until they are even with your shoulders, and then do five (5) sets of ten (10) reps w/increase in weight for each set.

Hamstrings - Five (5) sets, of ten (10) reps w/increase in weight for each set

Legs Curls (Hamstring Machine)

Lie flat on your stomach and place your legs underneath the pad at the end of the machine. Make sure that your heels fit comfortably on the pad, and then bring your legs up so that the pad touches the back of your buttocks. Next, do 5 sets of 10 reps w/increase in weight until you cannot get 10 reps, and then decrease the weight back down to get to reps.

Abdominals (Upper, Middle and Lower)

Always remember to do abs everyday and rotate whichever one you have not done; example: _If you do the upper abs on day one (1) then on day two (2) do the middle and on day three (3) do the lower abs; but on day four (4) go back and do the upper abs, finishing off with lower abs on day five (5)._

THE ARMOR OF GOD

FITNESS & TRAINING PROGRAM

extent. Do five (5) sets of ten (10) reps w/<u>increase</u> in weight for each set.

Calves – Five (5) sets, of ten (10) reps w/increase in weight for each set

Standing Calf Raises (Calf Machine)

For proper positioning of your body, first place your shoulders comfortably between the pads on the machine; then position your feet shoulder-width apart so most of your foot is on the rubber pad.

Keeping your knees locked, lower your heels so your toes stick up straight as you raise up on your feet; but make sure they are flat before you raise completely up as far as you can go towards the top on the soles of your feet. Do five (5) sets of ten (10) reps w/<u>increase</u> in weight for each set.

Seated Calf Raises (Hammer-Strength)

For proper positioning of your body, place feet shoulder-width apart and make sure the soles of your feet are comfortably on the bottom pad of machine.

Next, lift your feet up and release the lever so the pad rests comfortably on your knees. Do five (5) sets of ten (10) reps w/<u>increase</u> in weight for each set.

Abdominals (Upper, Middle and Lower)

Always remember to do abs everyday and rotate whichever one you have not done; example: *If you do the upper abs on day one (1) then on day two (2) do the middle and on day three (3) do the lower abs; but on day four (4) go back and do the upper abs, finishing off with lower abs on day five (5).*

THE ARMOR OF GOD

FITNESS & TRAINING PROGRAM

Phase Three: Power—Six (6) Weeks

The Word of God says; "The Lord hasn't given me the spirit of fear, but of <u>power</u>, love and a sound mind." (2 Tim. 1:7)

Five (5) days on, two (2) days off. One (1) body part per day and between each set, taking up to a two (2) five (5) minute rest period.

Make sure you drink plenty of water after each set *(at least one gallon per day)*. With this phase, you should already know what you could lift for eight (8) reps. After your first set of eight (8) reps, go straight to your maximum weight on each of the next sets to follow.

Day One (1) — Cardio, Chest and Abs

Cardio – 30 Minutes (Treadmill)

See example in phase one (1), day one (1)

<u>*Chest – Five (5) sets of eight (8) reps w/increase to maximum weight on each set*</u>

Incline Bench Press (Barbell)

For proper positioning of your body, lie flat on your back, keeping it straight as you sit firmly with your buttocks against the seat. For proper positioning for your hands, place them on the outside of the lines on the bar; then lift it off the rack. Lower the bar towards your chest so it touches the bottom of your neck and the top of your chest. Next, do five (5) sets of eight (8) reps w/<u>increase</u> in weight to your maximum.

THE ARMOR OF GOD
FITNESS & TRAINING PROGRAM

Decline Bench Press (Barbell)

For proper positioning of your body, sit down and place your feet underneath the pads on the front of the bench; then lift it off the rack. Lower the bar towards your chest so it touches the bottom of your chest and the top of your abs. Next, do five (5) sets of eight (8) reps w/<u>increase</u> in weight to your maximum.

Seated Incline Press (Hammer-Strength)

For proper positioning of the seat, adjust it so when you sit down on the seat, the bar almost touches your neck. Using your thumbs as a guide, place them at the very end of the bar where the rubber begins and then stretch out your hand to get a measurement. As you push the bar forward, make sure your back is firmly against the seat; then do set five (5) sets of eight (8) reps w/<u>increase</u> in weight to your until you cannot get eight (8) reps then, <u>decrease</u> the weight back down to get eight (8) reps.

Seated Decline Press (Hammer-Strength)

For proper positioning of the seat, adjust it so when you sit down on the seat and raise your arms up, the bar touches your shoulders evenly. Using your thumbs as a guide, place them at the very end of the bar where the rubber begins; then stretch out your hand to get a measurement. As you push the bar forward, make sure your back is firmly against the seat; then do five (5) sets of eight (8) reps w/<u>increase</u> in weight until you cannot get eight (8) reps, then <u>decrease</u> the weight back down to get eight (8) reps.

THE ARMOR OF GOD

FITNESS & TRAINING PROGRAM

Abdominals *(Upper, Middle and Lower)*

Always remember to do abs everyday and rotate whichever one you have not done; for example: If you do upper abs on day one (1) then on day two (2) do the middle, and on day three (3) the lower abs. But on day four (4), go back to the upper abs and on day five (5) finish with the lower abs.

Day Two (2) – Cardio, Back and Abs

Cardio – 30 Minutes (Treadmill)

See example in phase one (1), day one (1)

Back – Five (5) sets, eight (8) reps w/increase to maximum weight on each set

T-Bar Rows (Hammer-Strength)

For proper positioning of your body, stand firmly with your feet placed so the strongest is in the front of the other. Next, place your hands at the very end of the rubber on the bar, now pull the bar as close to you as possible without hitting the bottom of the bench, then do five (5) sets of eight (8) reps w/<u>increase</u> in weight until you cannot get eight (8) reps then, decrease the weight back down to get eight (8) reps.

Low Pulley Rows (Hammer-Strength)

Adjust your seat so when you sit down, your chin is touching the top of the seat. For proper positioning of your hands, place them on the bottom half of the curve on the bar. As you pull the weight towards you, sit up straight in the seat so your chest is flat against it, then do five (5) sets of eight (8) reps w/<u>increase</u> in weight until you cannot get eight (8) reps then, <u>decrease</u> the weight back down to get eight (8) reps.

THE ARMOR OF GOD
FITNESS & TRAINING PROGRAM

Pull Downs (Cable Machine)

For proper positioning of the machine, adjust the seat so the top part of your chest is even with the top part of the seat. For proper positioning of your hands, place them on the bottom half of the curve on the bar. Sit down, sit up straight and adjust the pads that fit on your legs with your knees. As you begin to pull the weight towards you, make sure you pull it so the bar is even with the bottom part of your chest, then do five (5) sets of eight (8) reps w/increase in weight until you cannot get eight (8) reps, then decrease weight back down to get eight (8) reps.

Dead lifts (Barbell)

For proper positioning of your hands, place your strongest hand reverse on the outside of the line on the bar, and the other hand frontward on the opposite outside line on the bar. For proper positioning of your feet, stand shoulder-width apart and squat down in a seated position and using your legs, push up and pull the bar so as you start to bend backwards, the bar passes your knees. Do five (5) sets of eight (8) reps w/increase in weight until you cannot get eight (8) reps, then decrease weight back down to get eight (8) reps.

Abdominals (Upper, Middle and Lower)

Always remember to do abs everyday and rotate whichever one you have not done; for example: *If you do upper abs on day one (1) then on day two (2) do the middle, and on day three (3) the lower abs; but on day four (4), go back to the upper abs and on day five (5) finish with lower abs.*

THE ARMOR OF GOD

FITNESS & TRAINING PROGRAM

Day Three (3) – Cardio, Legs (Quads, Hamstrings & Calves) and Abs

Cardio – 30 Minutes (Treadmill)

See example in phase one (1), day one (1)

Legs – (Quads, Hamstrings & Calves), Five (5) sets, eight (8) reps w/ increase in weight to maximum on each set

Squats (Barbell)

Go underneath the bar and place your neck evenly between the openings on the bar. After doing this, place your hands on the outside lines of the bar to balance it once you have lifted it from the rack, and using your legs, push up and take two (2) steps back-ward to clear the rack so that you don't have trouble squatting. Next, for proper positioning of your feet, place them shoulder-width apart to distribute your weight evenly. Lower your body to a seated position and then do five (5) sets of eight (8) reps w/<u>increase</u> in weight until you cannot get eight (8) reps, then <u>decrease</u> weight back down to get eight (8) reps.

Seated Incline Leg Press (Hammer-Strength)

For proper positioning of the machine, adjust the seat to the last position on the bench until it's almost flat, then sit down, lie flat on your back. Place your feet shoulder-width apart so they are touching the very top part of the rubber. Bring your legs down so they touch your chest, then do five (5) sets of eight (8) reps w/<u>increase</u> in weight until you cannot get eight (8) reps, then <u>decrease</u> weight back down to get eight (8) reps.

THE ARMOR OF GOD

FITNESS & TRAINING PROGRAM

Hack Squats (Hammer-Strength)

For proper positioning of your body, adjust yourself so the pads fit comfortably on your shoulders; place your feet shoulder-width apart so they are touching the very top of the machine. Next, lower yourself down as though you were sitting and do five (5) sets of eight (8) reps w/<u>increase</u> in weight until you cannot get eight (8) reps, then <u>decrease</u> weight back down to get eight (8) reps.

Leg Extensions (Cable Machine)

For proper positioning of your feet, place them underneath the pad at the bottom of the machine, shoulder-width apart. Next, bring your legs up so they come to an upright (vertical) position, and do five (5) sets of eight (8) reps w/<u>increase</u> in weight until you cannot get eight (8) reps, then <u>decrease</u> weight back down to get eight (8) reps.

Hamstrings – Five (5) sets, eight (8) reps w/increase in weight to maximum on each set

Leg Curls (Hamstring Machine)

Lying flat on your stomach, place your legs underneath the pad at the end of the machine so your heels fit comfortably under the pad. Bring your legs up so they touch the back of your buttocks and do five (5) sets of eight (8) reps w/<u>increase</u> in weight until you cannot get eight (8) reps, then <u>decrease</u> weight back down to get eight (8) reps.

Calves – Five (5) sets, eight (8) reps w/increase in weight to maximum on each set

THE ARMOR OF GOD

FITNESS & TRAINING PROGRAM

Standing Calf Raises (Calf Machine)

For proper positioning of your body, place your shoulders comfortably between the pads on the machine. For proper positioning of your feet, place them shoulder-width apart so most of your foot is on the rubber pad. Keeping your knees locked, lower your heels so the toes on your feet stick straight up as you rise up on the balls of your feet; make sure they are in a flat position before you raise completely up as far as you can on the balls of your feet. Next, do five (5) sets of eight (8) reps w/<u>increase</u> in weight until you cannot get eight (8) reps, then <u>decrease</u> weight back down to get eight (8) reps.

Abdominals (Upper, Middle and Lower)

Always remember to do abs everyday and rotate whichever one you have not done; for example: If you do upper abs on day one (1) then on day two (2) do the middle, and on day three (3) the lower abs; but on day four (4), go back to the upper abs and on day five (5) finish with lower abs.

Day Four (4) – Cardio, Shoulders and Abs

Cardio – 30 Minutes (Treadmill)

See example in phase one (1), day one (1)

Shoulders – Five (5) sets, eight (8) reps w/increase in weight to maximum on each set

THE ARMOR OF GOD

FITNESS & TRAINING PROGRAM

Seated Shoulder Press (Hammer-Strength)

Adjust the seat so bar is even with the top part of your chest; then sit down with your back firmly against the seat so your back is straight. For proper positioning of your hands, place thumbs at the tip of the rubber in the bar and stretch them out to grip the bar. Pushing upward, do five (5) sets of eight (8) reps w/<u>increase</u> in weight until you cannot get eight (8) reps; then <u>decrease</u> weight back down to get eight (8) reps.

Shoulder Shrugs (Barbell)

For proper positioning of your body, stand evenly between the open spaces on the bar and position your hands so your grip is even with the outside of your legs. Place your chin on your chest, keeping your arms firmly at your side and lift your shoulders up as far as they can go; as if you were shrugging your shoulders to say, *"I don't know?"* Do five (5) sets of eight (8) reps w/<u>increase</u> in weight until you cannot get eight (8) reps; then <u>decrease</u> the weight back down to get eight (8) reps.

Side Lateral Raises (Dumbbell)

For proper positioning of your body, stand with your feet shoulder-width apart as you hold the dumbbells against your body. Now begin to raise them so they are stretched out evenly with your shoulders. Next, do five (5) sets of eight (8) reps w/<u>increase</u> in weight until you cannot get eight (8) reps; then <u>decrease</u> the weight back down to get eight (8) reps.

THE ARMOR OF GOD

FITNESS & TRAINING PROGRAM

Seated Rear-Delt (Hammer-Strength)

For proper positioning of the machine, adjust the seat so you are sitting with your chest against the back of the seat, and your chin is on the top of the pad. Next, adjust the machine to the last forward position, then grip the ends of the rubber on the bar; and open your arms until they are even with your shoulders. Do five (5) sets of eight (8) reps w/<u>increase</u> in weight until you cannot get eight (8) reps; then <u>decrease</u> the weight back down to get eight (8) reps.

Abdominals (Upper, Middle and Lower)

Always remember to do abs everyday and rotate whichever one you have not done; for example: If you do upper abs on day one (1) then on day two (2) do the middle, and on day three (3) the lower abs; but on day four (4), go back to the upper abs and on day five (5) finish with lower abs.

Day Five (5) – Cardio, Arms (Triceps & Biceps) and Abs

Cardio – 30 Minutes (Treadmill)

See example in phase one (1), day one (1)

Triceps – Five (5) sets, eight (8) reps w/increase in weight to maximum on each set

THE ARMOR OF GOD

FITNESS & TRAINING PROGRAM

Close-Grip Bench Press (Barbell)

Laying down flat on your back, place your hands on each side of the bar where the grooves begin. Next, lift the bar off the rack and bring it down to the bottom edge of your chest. Push the bar so it's moving forward; then do five (5) sets of eight (8) reps w/<u>increase</u> in weight to maximum until you cannot get eight (8) reps; then <u>decrease</u> weight back down to get eight (8) reps.

Tricep Extensions (EZ Curl Bar)

Lie down on your back, and grip the curl bar in the middle on the inside of the curve. Slide down on the bench so the back of your head touches and you can see right in front of you. Next, place the bar on your chin and then do five (5) sets of eight (8) reps w/<u>same</u> weight for each set. For example:

Set One (1): Start at the chin.

Set Two (2): Go to the eyes.

Set Three (3): Go to the forehead.

Set Four (4): At the back of the head.

Set Five (5): Start at the back of the head and push out.

Tricep Pull Downs (Cable Machine)

Attach the small T-Shaped bar on the cable and for proper positioning of your feet, stand shoulder-width apart and grip the bar all the way at the end. Pull cable down so your arms are fully extended and as the weight takes your arms back up, <u>STOP;</u> to form the letter "L". Do five (5) sets of eight (8) reps w/<u>increase</u> in weight until you cannot get eight (8) reps; then <u>decrease</u> the weight back down to get eight (8) reps.

THE ARMOR OF GOD

FITNESS & TRAINING PROGRAM

Biceps – Five (5) sets, eight (8) reps w/increase in weight for each set

Standing Curls (Barbell)

For proper positioning of your feet, stand shoulder-width apart and place your hands on the outside lines of the bar for proper grip. Next, raise the bar so it reaches your chin without lowering your head, and then do five (5) sets of eight (8) reps w/<u>increase</u> in weight until you cannot get eight (8) reps; then <u>decrease</u> weight back to get eight (8) reps .

Seated Curls (Hammer-Strength)

Adjust seat, and placing your arms over the bench; your armpits should be on top of the pad making your arms stretch forward. For proper positioning of your hands, grip the attached bar where the rubber ends, and then pull the bar so it reaches your face.

Do five (5) sets of eight (8) reps w/increase in weight until you cannot get eight (8) reps; then decrease weight back down to get eight (8) reps.

Standing Dumbbell Curls (Dumbbells)

For the proper positioning of your body, place hands with dumbbells on the side of your body with weights facing outward. Next, place feet shoulder-width apart and raise dumbbells up one at a time towards your chest twisting hands so that your knuckles are facing straight ahead. Only raise the weights as far as your chin and use your arms not your shoulders. Do five (5) sets of eight (8) reps w/<u>increase</u> in weight until you cannot get eight (8) reps; then <u>decrease</u> weight back down to get eight (8) reps.

THE ARMOR OF GOD

FITNESS & TRAINING PROGRAM

<u>*Abdominals (Upper, Middle and Lower)*</u>

Always remember to do abs everyday and rotate whichever one you have not done; for example: If you do upper abs on day one (1) then on day two (2) do the middle, and on day three (3) the lower abs; but on day four (4), go back to the upper abs and on day five (5) finish with lower abs.

<u>*The Digestive System*</u>

The digestive systems' function is to break the food down into smaller molecules that the cells can use. Digestion begins in the mouth as food is mixed with saliva which contains enzymes that help break down carbohydrates and then it travels down the esophagus to the stomach where it's mixed with hydrochloric acid and several enzymes that digest protein. Located at the stomach is a round sphincter muscle that opens periodically, briefly letting food enter the intestines and thus the stomach becomes a storage for food as well as a digestive span as the food passes into the <u>*Small Intestines*</u>. The small intestines contain enzymes that help digest <u>*proteins*</u>, <u>*fats*</u> & <u>*carbohydrates*</u>, and are the main site for absorption of digested food into the bloodstream.

They are then carried by the blood to the cells that will use some of the nutrients and store the excess as <u>*glycogen*</u>, <u>*protein*</u>, or <u>*fat*</u>. These reserves are converted into <u>*glucose*</u>, the body's primary fuel, which is mobilized into the bloodstream and into the large intestine as water and minerals are absorbed while lubricating the remaining materials, passing them as feces.

THE ARMOR OF GOD

FITNESS & TRAINING PROGRAM

Enzymes & Consumption of Dairy Products

After a certain age, most mammals lose their ability to metabolize _lactose (the sugar in milk)_ because of declining levels of the intestinal enzyme _lactase_. From then on, consumption of milk can cause _gas_, _stomach cramps_, or _other signs of distress_, and the declining levels of lactase may be an evolved mechanism to encourage weaning at the appropriate times; for example: Humans are the exception because adults consume milk, cheese, ice cream and other products derived from cows & goats, but worldwide most adults cannot comfortably tolerate large amounts of milk products because _two-thirds (2/3)_ of all adults have low levels of lactase because of a recessive gene.

How Taste & Digestion Control Hunger

Oral Factors

1. People eat partly for the sake of taste.

2. Eating is also sustained by other facial sensations.

3. The tactile sensations are conveyed to the brain via the fifth (5th) cranial nerve (trigeminal nerve)

4. Taste and other oral sensations contribute to the regulation of eating, but they are not sufficient by themselves.

THE ARMOR OF GOD

FITNESS & TRAINING PROGRAM

Stomach & Intestines

The stomach conveys satiety messages to the brain via the Vagues nerve and the *splanchic nerves*, but satiety depends on stomach distension because it's the Vagues nerve *(cranial nerve)* that conveys information about the stretching of the stomach in ways that provide a major basis for satiety. The *splanchic nerves* convey information about the nutrient content of the stomach carrying impulses from the *thoracic and lumbar parts of the spinal cord to the digestive organs and from the digestive organs to the spinal cord*. The duodenum is part of the small intestine adjoining the stomach and is the first digestive site that absorbs a significant amount of nutrients, which causes the duodenum to release hormones with a satiating effect called Cholecystokinin (CCK). CCK decreases in size by closing the sphincter muscle between the stomach or duodenum causing the stomach to fill more quickly than it would have, and it is also a neurotransmitter in the brain, and it doesn't cross the blood or brain barrier in significant quantities.

Tip: Eating sugars have a quick satiating effect, but while the fats produce only weak sensations of satiety only after they are digested several hours, and the results are that most of the Body of Christ on these high-fat diets tend to overeat.

Blood Glucose

Glucose is digested food that enters the blood stream and is very important source of energy for all parts of the body, and it's the most important fuel of the brain. Some Theorist propose that the supply of glucose to the cells is the primary basis for hunger and satiety because availability of glucose to the cells can vary significantly as a function of changes in blood levels of two pancreatic hormones *Insulin & Glucagon*.

THE ARMOR OF GOD

FITNESS & TRAINING PROGRAM

Insulin facilitates the entry of glucose into the cells, which may either use the glucose for current energy needs or store it as *fat* or *glycogen*.

Glucagon has the reverse effect as insulin, and it stimulates the liver to convert stored glycogen to glucose thus raising blood glucose levels. How it works is after a meal, insulin levels rise causing much glucose to enter the cell and as time passes the blood glucose levels fall as the appetite decreases, but as the pancreas releases more glucagons and less insulin, then hunger returns; but when insulin levels are high, hunger is low because the blood is supplying the cells with glucose, and if the insulin level remains high after the last meal, the body continues to move blood glucose into the cells while the liver cells and fat cells continue to store it as glycogen; and consequently as the available blood glucose begins to decline, people with chronically high insulin levels tend to eat more and gain weight, but when the insulin level is extremely low, as is people with diabetes, blood glucose levels may exceed triple the normal level, so they eat more than usual because their cells are starving; but they lose weight Because the glucose is unavailable for energy and the fat cells are broken down. People produce more insulin both when they eat and getting ready to eat, which prepares the body to let more glucose enter the cells and store the excess as fats. Obese people produce more insulin causing more of their food to be stored as fat, which makes their appetite return sooner after a meal.

Hypothalamus & Feeding Regulations

The <u>Lateral Hypothalamus</u> is an important area for the control of feeding (*contributes in several ways*). First, the <u>Axon</u> from the <u>Lateral Hypothalamus</u> (*LH*) extends to the <u>Nucleus of the Tractus Solitarius</u> (*NTS*) in the medulla, and how it works is information from the *LH* modifies activity of some of the *NTS* cells by either altering the tastes sensation or by increasing the salvation response of tastes, which then activates a circuit that excites <u>dopamine</u> containing cells initiating and reinforcing learned behaviors. Then <u>Axons</u> from the *LH* extend into several forebrain structures facilitating ingestions, swallowing and causing cortical cells to increase responses to the <u>taste</u>, <u>smell</u>, and <u>texture of food</u>, while stimulating the release of insulin by the pancreas and digestive juices in the stomach.

<u>Genetics, Neurotransmitter & Feeding Regulation</u>

Your food choices and genes play a major role in a person's metabolic rate; bodyweight and genetics because your genes can control bodyweight and metabolic rate in people whose bodies produced more heat while maintaining low weight then those whose bodies metabolic rate generated less heat, conserve it better and gained weight without overeating. There's a protein that your fat cells produce called <u>Leptin</u>, and it circulates throughout the blood notifying the rest of the body about fat supplies, and the higher <u>Leptin</u> levels, then your hunger decreases.

<u>Boosting the Immune System with Herbs</u>

For over four thousand *(4,000)* years, the Chinese have used certain herbs to prevent common diseases. The ancient Chinese knew nothing of bacteria or viruses, yet some of the herbs were said to *"strengthen the exterior"*, or to *"shield"*.

Modern scientific research is confirming they were right. Thousands of years later, and 60 (sixty) years after the discovery of <u>penicillin</u>, the study of herbs affecting the immune system is one of the hottest topics in pharmacological research. Can herbs really strengthen our resistance and help us lead healthier lives? Both the wisdom of centuries of observation, and the scrutiny of the scientific laboratory, supports this view. Our immune system recognizes and destroys anything foreign to the body, including cells like bacteria and other microbes, and foreign particles including toxic compounds.

Cells in the circulatory and the lymphatic systems perform this recognition and destruction. These cells are produced in the bone marrow and lymphatic tissue (thymus, lymph nodes, spleen and tonsils) respectively. The cells begin their lives as *"stem cells"*, and they are so featureless that there is no way to determine what type of blood cell they will ultimately become. They may develop into any of a number of different kinds of cells, for instance: *red blood cells, various types of white blood cells, etc.* These cells are then released into the blood stream and are carried to all parts of the body, but there are essentially two types of cells, one of which is called *"memory cells"*. Memory cells, as the name implies, remember specific foreign cells or chemicals to which they have been exposed, and react immediately when they are next exposed to those compounds. Drugs that affect the memory cells stimulate immunity only to one disease or antigen, and vaccines are an example of drugs that effect memory cells. Most herbs for the immune system don't affect memory cells, but are general immune system stimulators *(immunostimulants)*. They increase the activity of the immune system but are not specific to a particular disease or *"antigen" (a protein against which immune cells act)*, but rather they increase resistance by mobilizing *"effector cells"* which act against all foreign particles rather than just one specific type *(i.e. a measles virus)*.

Remarkably, since the discovery of penicillin, our scientists, in search of drugs against infectious disease, have looked only for chemicals which kill bacteria or viruses, but finally they are coming to realize it is possible to boost the immune system, which can then fight naturally against infectious agents without the drawbacks of antibiotic therapy;

THE ARMOR OF GOD

FITNESS & TRAINING PROGRAM

but while immune stimulants cannot replace antibiotics in some cases, they have proven far superior in others. Here are a few of the best-researched immune boosters available in the health food stores:

Astragalus

The Chinese <u>Astragalus Root</u> or <u>Astragalus Membranaceus,</u> is widely used throughout the Orient as a tonic food and medicinal plant, and in Asia, this plant is sold as dried slices of root, six *(6)* to twelve *(12)* inches long. Research has shown that this root and its extracts are powerful stimulators of the immune system, and in Asia, the roots are frequently boiled along with other herb ingredients, mostly in chicken broth to produce a tonic/ medicinal soup, and has been used for thousands of years in China. First mentioned in the *Divine Husbandman's Classic of the Materia Medica,* an ancient Chinese medicinal text, Astragalus is said to *"tonify the spleen, blood and Qi"*, and is used for *"wasting and thirsting syndrome"*. Some of the specific Chinese uses hint at a stimulant effect on the immune system, for example: *it is used as a* tonic for the lungs, for frequent colds or shortness of breath, and the Chinese also use it internally for chronic ulcerations and other persistent external infections. Astragalus stimulates virtually every phase of immune system activity and it increases the number of "stem cells" in the marrow and lymph tissue and also stimulates their development into active immune cells that are then released into the body. Research documenting this also demonstrated that Astragalus could promote or trigger immune cells from the "resting" state into heightened activity.

THE ARMOR OF GOD

FITNESS & TRAINING PROGRAM

Another study on an *Astagalus-based* Chinese remedy demonstrated *"the tendency to stimulate immune response"* without suppressive effects and that *long-term* use *(365 days)* heightened the activity of the *spleen cells.* The remedy also decreased negative side effects of steroid therapy on the immune system, and the research recommends using it in combination with the steroid therapy *"to alleviate the adverse effects"* of the steroid. Perhaps the best evidence to date for the powerful immunostimulant effects of Astagalus come from the University of Texas Medical Center in Houston; there scientists tested damaged immune system cells from cancer patients and compared them against cells from the blood of normal human subjects. Astragalus extracts were able to completely restore the function of cancer patients' immune cells and in some cases the compromised cells were stimulated to greater activity than those from normal human subjects. The study concluded, *"Complete immune restoration can be achieved by using a fractionated extract of Astragalus Membranaceus, a traditional Chinese medicinal herb found to posses immune restorative activity in vitro".* Astragalus has also been found to stimulate the production of *Interferon,* which increases its effects in fighting disease. The combined effect of Interferon and Astragalus Root *"resulted not only in the decreased common cold incidence but also in shortening the course of illness. The average course of illness of the patients in the combined treatment group was 2.6 days as compared to 4.6 days in the controlled group."* In the same study, the Astragalus Root was found to *increase the life span* of human cells in culture studies and there was no toxicity to human cells. *"On the contrary, cell counts indicated that the vital cells in cultures treated with this drug for three (3) weeks were markedly more numerous than those without treatment and the treated cells also became* resistant to a common virus and the Astragalus Root promoted regeneration of cells in the Bronchi of virus-infected mice". As if this weren't impressive enough, another study probed the activity of <u>Macrophages</u> (one of the major cells responsible for consuming invading microbes), which significantly enhanced this activity within six (6) hours of treatment and the enhancement persisted for at least seventy-two (72) hours. The extract also significantly inhibited the growth of tumor cells in mice, especially when combined with the extract <u>Ligustrum Lucidum</u> *(pivet)*. The researchers remarked that Astragalus extract *"may thus restore immunocompetence and is potentially beneficial for cancer patients as well as AIDS patients"*. Most consumers probably use Astragalus Root to prevent and treat colds and other minor diseases, but in the Chinese research mentioned above, the Astragalus Root reduced the incidence of common colds among users and shortened the duration of colds by almost half.

Echinacea

This is a very popular American wildflower and garden plant, the purple coneflower. It's also one of America's most popular herbal products and is also used to prevent and treat the common cold; *influenza* and *infections*.

Echinacea is the best known and one of the most researched of all immunostimulants and was the most popular herb used by Native Americans; and at least fourteen (14) tribes used Echinacea for *coughs, colds, sore throats, infections, toothaches, inflammation, tonsillitis, snakebites, and other uses*, but were mostly used by the Dakotas as a veterinary medicine for their horses.

By the early twentieth (20th) century, Echinacea had become the best selling medicinal tincture in America, used for a variety of *internal* and *external* conditions; but by 1910 it had been dismissed as worthless by the <u>American Medical Association</u> *(AMA)* and although it continued to be used, Echinacea fell into disuse in this country by 1930. However, *Europeans* began growing and using Echinacea, especially the *Germans* and to this day have produced the best scientific documentation of its value.

THE ARMOR OF GOD

FITNESS & TRAINING PROGRAM

The extract's popularity in the U.S. grew rapidly during the 1980's and the plant is now again among America's best-selling herb extracts. The most common anecdotal reports about the use of Echinacea are from people who began to take the extract at the first sign of a cold, and often to their surprise, they find the cold had disappeared, usually within twenty-four (24) hours, and sometimes after taking the extract only once; but anecdotal evidence carries little weight in scientific circles, but plant drug researches have conducted over three hundred and fifty (350) scientific studies about Echinacea, and here's what some of those studies say about Echinacea: *"The most consistently proven effect of Echinacea is in stimulating <u>phagocytosis</u> or the consumption of invading organisms by <u>white blood cells</u> and <u>lymphocytes"</u>.*

To prove this, scientists incubate human white blood cells, yeast cells and Echinacea extract, and then they examine the blood cells microscopically and count the number of yeast cells are gobbled up by the blood cells. Extracts of Echinacea can increase phagocytosis by 20 (twenty)—40 (forty) percent (%), and in another test called *"the carbon clearance test"*; it measures the speed of the carbon particles removed from the injected bloodstream of a mouse. The quicker the mouse can remove the injected foreign particles, means that more of its immune system has been stimulated; but also in this test, Echinacea extracts excel and thus confirming the fact that this remarkable plant increases the activity of the immune system cells so they can eliminate invading organisms and foreign particles more quickly. As with Astragalus, Echinacea causes an increase in the number of immune cells, further enhancing the overall activity of the immune system and also stimulates the production of *Interferon* as well as other important products of the immune system, including *"The Tumor Necrosis Factor"*, which is very important to the body's response against cancer.

THE ARMOR OF GOD
FITNESS & TRAINING PROGRAM

Echinacea also inhibits an enzyme *(Hyaluronidase)*, which is secreted by bacteria, and helps them gain access to healthy cells in the body, but researchers in the early 1950's showed that Echinacea could completely counteract the effect of this enzyme and this could help prevent infection when used to treat wounds, and while Echinacea is usually used internally for the treatment of *viruses* and *bacteria,* it is being used more externally for the treatment of wounds. It also kills yeast and slows the growth of bacteria and helps to stimulate the growth of new tissue as well as combating inflammation, further supporting its use in the treatment of wounds.

Research in 1957, showed that an extract of Echinacea caused a twenty-two (22) percent (%) reduction in inflammation among arthritis suffers, but that is only about half as steroids because they have serious side-effects. Steroids also strongly *suppress* the immune system, which makes them a poor choice for treating any condition in which infection is likely, while Echinacea on the other hand, a non-toxic; adds immune-stimulating properties to its anti-flammatory effect. Most people use Echinacea for warding off colds and influenza because extracts whether alcoholic or non-alcoholic, are the most commonly used forms and the usual amount taken is one (1) dropper-full at a time fifteen – twenty-five (15-25) drops. This is taken at the first sign of a cold and is repeated two (2) or three (3) times a day.

European clinics don't use continuous doses of Echinacea but rather alternate three (3) days on and three (3) days off because testing shows that the immune system in healthy subjects can only be stimulated briefly before returning back to its normal state, and after several days without stimulation, *immunostimulants* can again be effective. Echinacea has an excellent safety record because after hundreds of years of use, there is no toxicity or side effects reported, except rare allergic reactions in sensitive individuals.

THE ARMOR OF GOD

FITNESS & TRAINING PROGRAM

The purple coneflower is a truly American contribution to the world of health care through herbs, and this safe, effective immune stimulant was discovered and first used by the Native American and is now a major medicinal plant throughout Europe and the USA.

Astragalus & Echinacea References:

Bensky, D. and Gamble, A., Chinese Herbal Medicine, 1986, Eastland Press.

Rou, Ma and Ren Fu-Xie, Journal of Traditional Chinese Medicine, 1983, 3(3) pp. 199-204.

Iwama, H., et al., 1986, Planta Medicia, pp. 247-250.

Mavligit, G.M., et al., 1979, J. Immunology, 123, pp. 2185-2188.

Sun, Y., Cancer, 52(1), 1983, 7/3, pp. 70-73.

Chu, D., et al., Clin. Lab. Immuno., 1988, 25, 125-129.

Yunde, H., Chinese Medical Journal, 1981, 94 (1), pp. 35-40.

Lau, B., et al., Phytotherapy Research, 1989, 3(4), pp. 148-153.

Digestive System References:

Abrams, S., the Black Physique, 2000, 8(3), pp. 51-55.

THE ARMOR OF GOD

FITNESS & TRAINING PROGRAM

TRUST IN THE LORD

Psalm 91

"He who dwells in the secret place of the MOST HIGH shall remain stable and fixed under the shadow of the ALMIGHTY; whose power no foe can withstand. I shall say of the LORD, HE is my refuge and my fortress, my GOD, on HIM I lean and rely, and in HIM I confidently trust! For then HE shall deliver you from the snare of the fowler and from the deadly pestilence. Then HE shall cover you with HIS Feathers, and under HIS Wings shall you trust and find refuge; HIS Truth and HIS Faithfulness are a shield and a buckler. Then you shall not be afraid of the terror of the night, nor of the arrows; the evil plots and slanders of the wicked that flies by day, nor of the pestilence that stalks in darkness, nor of the destruction and sudden death that surprise and lay waste at noonday.

Then a thousand may fall at your side, and ten thousand at your right hand, but it shall not come near you. Only a spectator shall you be; yourself inaccessible in the secret place of the MOST HIGH as you witness the reward of the wicked. Because you have made the LORD your refuge, and the MOST HIGH your dwelling place, there shall no evil befall you, nor plague or calamity come near your dwelling. For HE will give HIS Angels special charge over you, to accompany and defend and preserve you in all your ways of obedience and service. They shall bear you up on their hands, lest you dash your foot against a stone. You shall tread upon the lion and cobra, the young lion and the serpent shall you trample under foot.

Because HE has set HIS Love upon ME, therefore I shall deliver him; I shall set him on high because he knows and understands MY Name; he has a personal knowledge of MY Mercy, Love and Kindness; trusts and relies on ME, knowing I shall never forsake him, no, never. He shall call upon ME, and I shall answer him; I shall be with him in trouble, I shall deliver him and honor him. With long life shall I satisfy him, and show him MY Mercy."

THE ARMOR OF GOD

FITNESS & TRAINING

LOG

Name		30 DAY	60 DAY	90 DAY	GOAL																		
Body Weight																							
Body Fat %																							
Measurements:																							
Shoulders																							
Chest																							
Waist																							
Hips																							
Thighs																							
Calves																							
Arms																							
Forearms